Paleo Diet
A Guide to Getting Started

Introduction

I want to thank you and congratulate you for purchasing the book, *"Paleo Diet: A Guide to Getting Started"*.

This book has actionable information on how to get started in the Paleo diet.

Humans got creative with food, and then the problem set in. Nature already provided us with all the foods we would need until the end of time. Even today, there are thousands of crops, fruits, sweeteners and condiments. These natural foods provided by nature are what our bodies are designed to process.

But somehow, we were not satisfied.

We decided to experiment a little, so we started cooking our foods and adding a little of this and that to create a more thrilling experience. We completely forgot that food wasn't a source of recreation and its only purpose is to provide the nutrients that our bodies need to function.

Eventually, in a bid to make money, some people discovered the art of processing and packaging food and selling them to people. But they also got greedy. In order to expand profits and create new products, they learned how to add some chemicals to the foods to make them sweeter, double up food quantities, or get people addicted to their products.

Soon enough, our feeding patterns deviated a lot from what was natural and what our bodies were designed to process. Our foods became very artificial and many of the preservatives and additives started poisoning our bodies.

Some researchers and nutritionists, after conducting several studies, discovered that the only way to save the human race from many of these new age diseases, which are mostly triggered by our diets, is to have us return to a natural diet; the one our bodies were designed to handle.

The Paleolithic diet is a diet that requires you to eat like the Paleolithic humans, our ancestors who lived during the Stone Age.

In this guide, you'll discover:

- What the Paleo diet is all about

- The health benefits of the Paleo diet

- The rules and principles of the diet

- A comprehensive list of what to eat and what to exclude from your diet

- A 7-day Paleo diet meal plan to help kick start your diet

- Delicious breakfast lunch and dinner recipes

- And much more!

If you are eager to make the most of the Paleo diet to transform your life for the better, this book is for you.

Thanks again for purchasing this book. I hope you enjoy it!

Chapter 1: That Time When There Were No Farms or Kitchens

Paleo is short for Paleolithic, a pre-start period of human development that existed over 2.5 million years ago. People who lived in the Paleolithic era were a species of archaic humans known as the Stone Age humans or the Homo erectus.

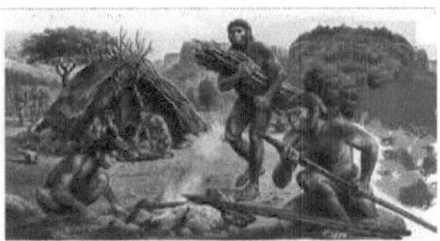

During the Paleolithic era, humans were yet to learn about agriculture or animal domestication. This meant that humans only ate foods that were readily available to them in their surrounding environment.

The humans who lived in this era were hunter-gatherers because they had to hunt for animals that they could eat, or pick up fruits, vegetables, fish, seeds, and nuts. There were no dairy products and they didn't eat grains or legumes because the hunter-gatherers didn't cook - there were no pots and cooking was a technological advancement that came much later.

The Stone Age humans adapted to this lifestyle, becoming genetically stronger and healthier by consuming more of these foods. They ate this way for more than 2 million years until the concept of agriculture was introduced, just about 10,000 years ago, and with agriculture came cooking, processing and preservation of foods.

Now, here is where the problem lies:

The human body is evolutionary in nature - our bodies are always growing and adapting to its changing surroundings and situations. As the environment in which we live in, and our lifestyles continue to change, the human body is always going through morphological, physiological, behavioral and developmental changes to cope with its current situations.

For instance, look at us today; many of us can barely step outside our homes when it's snowing and during the hot summer months, we can barely stay within our homes without air conditioning. But some 10,000 years ago, there was nothing like air conditioning and most humans only had leaves for clothes, there were no fancy duvets or blankets to keep them warm or hot water to shower but somehow, they survived. Because we now have access to all these technologies to make us comfortable, our bodies have now adapted to this level of comfort and the former way of living no longer feels comfortable. This is just one example of how the human body adjusts itself and adapts to current situations.

However, these adaptations don't happen overnight; it usually takes thousands or millions of years.

For instance, humans spent over 1.8 million years as Homo erectus before we evolved into our current state as Homo sapiens.

Now, we've only been Homo sapiens for about 300,000 years, which means that even though we are now Homo sapiens, our evolution is not complete, and we still have some of the characteristics of our Homo erectus ancestors.

What I am driving at is this - we spent 2.5 million years eating as hunter-gatherers and *boom!* 10,000 years ago, our diets change, and we start eating all these grains, legumes, dairy, and processed and preserved foods.

These foods are still new to humans and our bodies have not evolved enough to be able to digest and process them. Therefore, many of us are either overweight or in a constant struggle to maintain a healthy weight - our digestive system hasn't evolved enough to handle this 'strange diet'.

The human body takes a lot of time to readjust or adapt when you expose it to new concepts.

Have you ever been on a fast or restrictive diet? Or gone for a long period without food?

If you have, you'll notice that when you started to eat normally again, your stomach couldn't handle a lot of food. You may have even had some bloating, indigestion or constipation when you started trying to eat normally again. It probably took a while before your body was able to adjust to your former feeding pattern again. And of course, it depends on how long you were on the fast; the longer the fast lasted, the more time it would have taken for your body to adjust.

Or have you ever seen a person who was in a coma for a long time? Usually, when they come back to, they have to learn how to use their limbs and most of their body functions again.

Many of them will usually spend a lot of weeks in physiotherapy where they have to relearn how to use their limbs again.

That tells you how sensitive to changes the human body is. When you introduce the body to a new concept, after a period, your body adapts to it. But if you introduce another new concept or try to return it to a former concept, it will take also take a while before your body readjusts again.

Now, imagine eating a certain way for more than 2.5 million years, of course, it will take more than a meager 10,000 years to completely adapt to a new feeding pattern.

Our Diets are Evolving Faster than Our Bodies

There have been a lot of studies on human DNA that prove that the human genetic pattern has only changed by less than 0.02% in the last 40,000 years. This means that even though we can no longer be called Stone Age Humans, we still share a significant part of our DNAs. Our body systems are still pretty much the same.

Now, even though our bodies haven't changed so much, our diets have changed a lot.

The Stone Age human didn't drink milk because he didn't have the knowledge or skills to milk animals.

He did not eat domesticated animals like cows, sheep, and goats; neither did he consume meats from animals that have been fed with chemicals that are formulated to fatten them. If he wanted to eat meat, he had to hunt for animals in the wild, which were mostly lean meat and were very healthy.

He also didn't eat farmed eggs, hot dogs or processed or packaged meats.

The Paleolithic human never tasted grains or cereals and he never added any salt to his food.

He also had no access to refined sweeteners.

Let's look at our diet today; the average human diet today contains:

- 14% calories from dairy
- 31% of calories from cereals
- 4% of calories from candy, cake, cookies and other sweeteners
- 8% of calories from sodas, processed fruit juice and other beverages

- 4% calories from oils and dressings

- 39% calories from animal foods and derivatives

These foods are still very strange to the human body and they are upsetting the body and triggering the onset of many diseases including cancer, diabetes, obesity, depression, and many other health problems.

This means if we want to be as healthy as our Paleolithic ancestors, we must strive to eat as much as possible like the Paleo man. The Paleo diet strives to model that kind of diet. Let's discuss that next.

Chapter 2: What is The Paleo Diet?

The Paleo diet is basically a return to the status quo. It is a pattern of eating that mimics that of the Paleolithic human and it involves feeding the body with foods that it can process easily; foods that won't have you struggling to maintain a healthy weight or trigger diseases because your body cannot process them easily.

Basically, the Paleo diet is about eating the same types of foods that the Paleolithic human ate, and very little or no grains, legumes, processed foods, or any foods that didn't exist in the Paleolithic era.

The Paleolithic diet was first suggested by a gastroenterologist named Walter Voegtlin in the 1970's.

He suggested that by eating like our human ancestors, the Paleolithic human, can help to cure or significantly reduce incidences of a number of diseases including obesity, indigestion, diabetes, and Chron's disease.

He carried out an extensive research on the subject, and documented his findings in a book titled *"The Stone Age Diet: Based on an In-depth Studies of Human Ecology and the Diet of Man"*

Walter Voegtlin was also able to successfully treat a good number of patients suffering from different types of intestinal conditions and digestive problems by placing them on the Paleolithic diet.

In 1984, an Australian Doctor named Kerin O'Dea carried another study that backed up Walter Voegtlin's claims.

For the study, he placed a group of 10 Aborigines (Native Australians) who had been living as hunter-gatherers on a westernized diet. They were made to live in a nearby farming community and made to eat the same foods as the members of that community, including processed foods.

All of them became overweight, with many of them developing symptoms of Type 2 diabetes, high blood pressure, increased blood glucose and blood lipids.

They were then made to return to their previous hunter-gathering diet for a 7-week period and soon, within this period, all of these symptoms began to vanish, and they lost all the excess weight they had gained.

Another Doctor from Sweden carried out several studies over a 25-year period. Dr. Staffan Linberg M.D, PhD, of the Lund University, Sweden discovered that diets excluding dairy, cereals, vegetables oils, and cereals led to healthy aging.

He noted that older citizens who excluded these items from their diets over a 25-year period were mostly free from cardiovascular diseases, obesity, hypertension, diabetes, and cerebral conditions compared to others within the same age group who indulged in these foods.

However, it was another American Doctor, Dr. Loren Cordain who made the Paleo diet popular. Dr. Cordian, a professional nutritionist and physiologist, noted that many people were starving themselves in a bid to achieve healthy and lean bodies without much result.

This led him to carry out extensive research on the subject and eventually, he posited and demonstrated that a person can lose weight as well as prevent or reduce symptoms of several diseases like osteoporosis, heart diseases, metabolic syndrome, cancer and many other diseases just by sticking to a diet of fresh fruits, non-starchy vegetables, meat, fish, nuts, and other foods that the Stone Age humans ate.

Dr. Loren Cordan explained that by eating like the Paleolithic human, there will be no need for people to count calories, go on restrictive diets where they have to cut out carbs or other macronutrients from their diets, or starve themselves in order to maintain a healthy weight or body.

The aim of the Paleo diet is to eat like the Paleolithic humans who didn't engage in any type of farming hence didn't eat food groups that required farming, processing, or preservation of food with chemicals.

These foods, Dr. Cordan explains, are direct or indirect triggers of many of the new age diseases that are growing in popularity and ravaging the human body today.

Let's discuss some of the benefits that those following the Paleo diet have been able to obtain:

The Health Benefits of the Paleo Diet

1. **No More Chemical Ingestion**: Many of the foods that we eat today are laden with chemicals and additives that are designed to enhance food coloring, taste and shelf life. These additives mostly have no nutritional value other than to introduce toxins into your body. On the Paleo diet, you can't eat any processed foods or foods that bring chemicals to your body, as this is not allowed.

2. **You Eat More Nutrients**: You'll start using food for what it is meant for - to provide nutrients that your body needs and instead of eating foods that

are mostly bereft of nutrients, you'll start eating foods that contain a lot of vitamins and minerals that your body needs such as fruits, vegetables, healthy oils, nuts, and seeds.

3. **You Lose Weight**: The Paleo diet helps to improve gut health and metabolism; two factors that are very essential for weight loss. This is why a lot of people lose weight rapidly within the first few weeks on the diet.

   The increase in metabolic speed is due to the increased intake of Omega 3 and Omega 6 fatty acids from the healthy oils, wild-caught fishes and healthy nuts that you'll be consuming on the diet. Omega 3 and Omega 6 aids the body in burning fat.

   Increased intake of processed diary, oils and artificial sweeteners is one of the leading causes of poor gut health. Eliminating these foods from your diet helps to improve your gut health and subsequently, your weight.

4. **It Balances Your Blood Sugar Levels**: By eliminating the consumption of artificial food, sweeteners, grains, processed foods, drinks and baked goods, you automatically reduce your blood sugar. Most of the foods allowed on the Paleo diet also have very low Glycemic index so that the glucose is slowly released into your blood cells and as such will not cause sudden spikes in blood sugar.

   Fluctuations in blood sugar not only causes excessive food cravings, but also leads to insulin resistance, a condition where body cells become less responsive to insulin, the chemical messenger that is supposed to aid in the use of glucose.

5. **It Gives You a Healthy Skin**: The increase in Omega 3/6 fatty acids and saturated fats intake makes your skin healthier and brighter. Omega 3 and 6 fatty acids also improve brain function, especially contributing to enhanced mental clarity, mood and attitude.

So how exactly does the diet work? What rules are we supposed to adhere to while on the Paleo diet? That's what we will be discussing next.

Chapter 3: Rules of the Paleo Diet

The major rule of the Paleo diet is this - *If the Paleolithic man didn't eat it, don't eat it*.

It's as simple as that. However, to make it easier for you to master the rules and follow the diet, here is a breakdown of the rules.

If it's processed and packaged, don't eat it

Most processed and packaged foods contain chemical additives and preservatives that are potentially harmful to the human body. Some of these chemicals include Butylated Hydroxyanisole (BHA), Sodium Benzoate, shortening agents, and sodium nitrates. When you eat these foods, they cause a toxic build-up of these chemicals within your body and these toxins are potentially harmful to your body.

If it contains any ingredient you can't recognize or pronounce, don't eat it

Only eat foods with ingredients that you can identify.

If it was raised in a fishpond, don't eat it

Eat fish that grew in its natural habitat and avoid any type of farmed fish or sea food because most of the farmed fishes are fed with feeds that are heavily laden with chemicals and additives that are supposed to help boost their growth. These additives are potentially harmful to the body so when you consume them, you also ingest these toxins.

If it wasn't pasture raised, don't eat its meat or its egg

The same thing goes for meat; you should only eat meat from grass-fed, pasture-raised animals, or game meat hunted from the wild because farmed animals are also mostly fed with chemical laden feeds.

Don't Eat Grains and Legumes

You can't eat any grains or legumes on the Paleo diet because the Paleolithic humans didn't eat them. Most grains and legumes contain something called Gluten, a defensive chemical genetically developed by plants to stop predators from consuming them.

The human body cannot effectively digest and absorb gluten and when gluten is left to buildup in the body, it can trigger a number of autoimmune diseases.

Eat Fruits and Vegetables that are in Season

There are a lot of healthy fruits, roots and vegetables that are available for every season. Stick to eating in-season fruits and vegetables so that you can avoid eating heavily preserved, or genetically modified fruits and vegetables.

If you can, start your own garden.

Eat a Lot of Healthy Proteins and Fats

Make sure you eat a lot of healthy, Paleo-compliant proteins and fats as they contain a lot of the nutrients and minerals that your body needs to grow, thrive and stay healthy.

Below is a comprehensive list of foods that you can eat, and foods you should not eat on the Paleo diet.

What to Eat on the Paleo Diet

Pasture-raised meat	Pasture-raised goat, beef, lamb, pork, veal, bison, rabbit
Game Meat	Wild turkey, deer, reindeer, pheasant, rabbit, moose, boar, elk, woodcock
Wild Caught Fish	Flatfish, salmon, trout, tuna, catfish, anchovy, mackerel, herring, bass, tilapia, halibut, haddock, groupa, sole, turbot, walleye
Poultry	Free-range goose, chicken, duck, turkey, quail
Wild Caught Shellfish	Including oysters, clams, shrimps, mussels, crab, scallops, lobsters
Fats	Coconut milk, avocado, coconut flesh, avocado oil, ghee/clarified butter, tallow, olive oil, coconut oil, non-factory farmed fatty fishes including salmon, mackerel, sardines, veal fat, duck fat, lamb fat, walnut, macadamia, nut butters
Egg	Free-range eggs including goose eggs, chicken eggs, quail eggs and duck eggs
Fruits	Honeydew lemons, bananas, lychee, strawberry, raspberry, cranberry, blackberry, blueberry, oranges, apples, coconut, persimmon, pears, plantains, lime, olives, lemon, kiwi, passion fruit, dates, watermelon, figs, cantaloupe, apricot, cherries, grapes, pineapple, plantains, papaya, pomegranates, plums, grapefruits
Seeds and Nuts	Brazil nuts, sunflower seeds, flax seeds, pumpkin seeds/pepitas, pine nuts, hazel nuts, cashews, pecans, macadamia nuts, pistachios, chia seeds, walnuts, sesame seeds, almonds, chestnuts
Vegetables	**Vegetables**: Celery, broccoli, tomatoes, asparagus, bell peppers, cucumber, onions,

	cabbage, leeks, Brussels sprouts, kohlrabi, artichokes, green onions, eggplants, okra, cauliflower, avocados.
	Green Leafy Vegetables: Lettuce, watercress, spinach, turnip greens, collard greens, seaweeds, kale, endives, beet tops, mustard greens, arugula, dandelion, Swiss chard, bok choy, radicchio, chicory, rapini
	Root Vegetables: Carrots, cassava, yams, beets, turnips, parsnips, Jerusalem artichokes, rutabaga, radish, sweet potatoes
Squash	**Winter Squash:** Acorn squash, buttercup squash, butternut squash, pumpkin, spaghetti squash
	Summer Squash: Yellow summer squash, zucchini, crookneck squash
Mushrooms	Oyster, button, morel, portabella, porcini, shiitake, crimini, chanterelle
Herbs and Spices	Ginger, parsley, garlic, thyme, onions, lavender, black pepper, mint, hot peppers, basil, star anise, rosemary, fennel seeds, chives, mustard seeds, tarragon, cayenne pepper, oregano, cumin, turmeric, sage, cinnamon, dill, nutmeg, bay leaves, paprika, coriander, horseradish, vanilla, chilies, cloves
Seasonings/Condiments	Himalayan pink salt, sea salt, Homemade Mayo (made with egg yolk, mustard powder, salt, lemon juice, vinegar, and any Paleo compliant nuts), Mustard (made with soaked and blended mustard seeds with salt and vinegar), vinegar, lemon juice, any other Paleo branded condiment from a trusted supplier
Sweeteners	Date sugar, stevia, honey, monk fruit, blackstrap molasses, maple syrup, coconut sugar

Drinks and Others	Water, coconut water, mineral water, green tea, herbal teas, homemade fruit juice, almond or nut milk

What to Avoid On the Paleo Diet

Added Sugars and Artificial Sweeteners	Agave, sodas, baked goods, high fructose corn syrup, pastries, cane sugar, cane juice, fruit juice, aspartame
Legumes and Grains	Wheat, soybeans, barley, lentils, rye, pinto beans, oats, red beans, brown rice, peanuts, millet, chickpeas, spelt, bulgur wheat, couscous, kidney beans.
Processed Foods	All commercially packaged foods, any processed foods that contain additives that are not directly from nature.
Refined Vegetable Oils	Cottonseed oil, soybean oil, safflower oil, peanut oil, sunflower oil, corn oil, margarine, canola oil
Dairy or Products made with Dairy	Ice cream, milk, yoghurt, cheese
Drinks	Sodas, sweetened beverages, beer, drinks with artificial sweeteners

Now that you have a good understanding of what the Paleo diet is about, let's take our discussion a bit further where we talk about how to prepare different dishes with the allowed ingredients.

Chapter 3: Paleo Breakfast Recipes

Coconut Fruit Bowl

Ingredients

Serves 4

1 medium-sized fresh pineapples (diced)

4 ripe bananas (sliced)

1 ⅓ cups of full-fat coconut milk (chilled)

4 Navel oranges (peeled and cut in half)

¼ cup fresh lime juice

2 cups of seedless grapes (halved)

Garnish: Fresh mint leaves and shredded coconut

Directions

Combine all ingredients in a bowl then add mint leaves and shredded coconuts on top.

Serve chilled.

Coconut Berry Bowl

Ingredients

Serves 4

1 teaspoon of ginger (freshly grounded)

½ teaspoon of vanilla extract

Dash of cinnamon

2 cups of mixed berries (frozen)

Juice of 1 lemon

1 can of full-fat coconut milk

Directions

Combine coconut milk, lemon juice, vanilla extract, and fresh ginger in a bowl. Mix well.

Divide berries amongst serving bowls and pour coconut milk mix on top.

Sprinkle cinnamon over it and enjoy.

Salmon and Potato Pie

Ingredients

Serves 8 (includes 4 servings for next day)

4 tablespoons fresh chives (minced)

8 cups of salmon (cooked and shredded)

6 tablespoons of ghee

16 russet potatoes (peeled and sliced thinly)

2 tablespoons of tapioca starch

4 carrots (diced)

2 celery stalks (diced)

4 garlic cloves (minced)

Freshly ground black pepper to taste

Sea salt to taste

2 red onions (diced)

Directions

Start by preheating your oven to 375 degrees F.

Then place a saucepan over medium heat and add ghee to melt.

Pour tapioca starch in melted ghee and stir continuously.

Add coconut milk and continue to stir until it thickens.

Add seasoning.

Combine celery, salmon, onions, carrots, and chives in a bowl and add black pepper and sea salt to taste.

Add half of your potatoes to the bottom of a baking pan sprayed lightly with cooking spray.

Add half of the salmon and carrot mixture on top.

Add half of your tapioca sauce on top.

Pour the rest of your potatoes on top and pour the remaining tapioca starch and salmon mixture on top.

Bake in the oven for 45 minutes.

Serve half and preserve half for breakfast the next day.

Eggs in Sweet Potato Nests

Ingredients

Serves 8 (including servings for the next day)

24 free-range eggs

Ghee (melted)

8 sweet potatoes

4 tablespoons fresh chives (minced)

12 slices of bacon (cooked and crumbled)

Freshly ground pepper to taste

Sea salt to taste

Directions

Pre-heat your oven to 400 degrees F.

Bake sweet potatoes in the oven for 35 minutes and allow it cool down afterwards.

Peel and grate potatoes.

Add 3 tablespoons of grated potato into 24 muffin cups.

Make a nest shape in each muffin cup with your fingers and break one egg each into the nest.

Add salt and black pepper to taste.

Add fresh chives on top.

Bake until eggs set.

Serve with grilled bacons on the side.

Eggs Benedict and Ham

Ingredients

Serves 4

1 tablespoon of white wine vinegar

8 thin slices of ham

¼ cup of extra virgin olive oil

8 large eggs

1 teaspoon of lemon juice

Freshly ground black pepper to taste

Sea salt to taste

4 cups of hollandaise sauce

1 red bell pepper (thinly sliced)

Directions

Start by preheating the oven to 350 degrees F.

Cut each slice of ham from the center to the side to open it up.

Line a muffin tray with each ham slice to make the ham slices look like a cupcake wrapper.

Crack eggs into each ham-lined muffin cup.

Add black pepper and sea salt to taste.

Bake in the oven for 15 minutes.

Place a saucepan over medium heat and add olive oil to heat up.

Add red pepper and sauté for 3 minutes until crunchy.

To make vinaigrette, combine white wine vinegar, hollandaise sauce, and lemon juice in a bowl; whisk to combine.

Add black pepper and sea salt to taste.

Combine cooked red bell pepper with Arugula. Divide among serving plates and add vinaigrette on top.

Add 2 egg and ham cups on top of each dish.

Serve with some hollandaise sauce drizzled on top.

Chapter 4: Paleo Lunch Recipes

Root Vegetable Bowls with Cinnamon Maple and Tahini Dressing

Ingredients

Serves 4

For Root Vegetable Buddha Bowls:

3 cups of cooked brown rice

2 medium gold beets (peeled and cut into wedges)

1 large sweet potato (peeled and then chopped)

2 large parsnips (peeled and then chopped)

½ of a small cabbage (sliced)

10 ounces spinach

Sea salt to taste

Olive oil for roasting

For Maple Cinnamon Tahini Dressing:

¼ teaspoon of salt

2 ¼ cups of Tahini

1 tablespoon of fresh lemon juice

½ teaspoon ground cinnamon

¼ cup of water

2 tablespoons of pure maple syrup

Directions

Start by preheating the oven to 375 degrees F.

Combine root vegetables in a bowl and mix nicely.

Grease two baking sheets lightly with olive oil and divide root vegetables amongst the baking sheets.

Drizzle olive oil on the vegetables and add black pepper and sea salt.

Place in the oven to roast for 35 minutes or until slightly browned.

Combine Maple Tahini dressing ingredients in your blender and process until smooth.

Divide cooked brown rice, spinach and cabbage among serving dishes.

Add roasted root vegetables to the serving bowls.

Add desired amount of Maple Tahini dressing on top.

Enjoy.

Salad Nicoise

Ingredients

Serves 4

For Salad:

¼ cups of nicoise olives

16 ounces of grilled tuna steak

1 tablespoon of capers (rinsed)

4 hard-boiled eggs (peeled and sliced)

8 ounces green beans (cooked with ends trimmed)

2 Boston lettuce leaves (washed)

1 small red onion (diced)

3 small ripe tomatoes (cored and sliced into eights)

Freshly ground black pepper to taste

Sea salt to taste

For Vinaigrette:

1 teaspoon Dijon sauce

½ cup lemon juice

2 teaspoon of fresh oregano leaves (minced)

¾ cups of extra virgin olive oil

1 tablespoons of fresh thyme (minced)

2 tablespoons fresh basil leaves (minced)

1 medium shallot (minced)

Freshly ground black pepper to taste

Sea salt to taste

Directions

Combine ingredients for vinaigrette in a bowl and whisk to combine.

Combine salad ingredients in a bowl and mix well.

Divide salad among serving dishes and drizzle vinaigrette on top.

Garnish with capers.

Slow-Cooker Brisket Taco Bowls

Ingredients

Serves 4

For Taco Bowls:

As much greens as you want (spinach, lettuce, kale)

Guacamole

Lime wedges

Hot sauce

Olives

Quick pickled red onions and radishes

Segmented orange slices

For Brisket:

¼ teaspoon of ground ginger

2 lbs. beef brisket

1 ½ cups of orange juice

1 large onion (chopped)

½ cup of beef broth

6 cloves of garlic (minced)

1 inch-sized piece of ginger

Granulated garlic, black pepper and sea salt to taste

Juice and zest of 1 lime

½ teaspoon of cumin

¼ teaspoon of cinnamon

¼ teaspoon of cloves

Directions

Combine garlic and chopped onions in the bottom of a slow cooker.

Then nestle beef briskets on top of garlic and onions.

Add salt, pepper and granulated garlic to both sides of the brisket.

Sprinkle cinnamon, cumin, ground ginger and cloves inside the pot.

Add lime juice and zest.

Cook on low heat for 6-8 hours.

Combine taco bowl ingredients.

Serve with beef briskets on top.

Low-Carb Paleo Zucchini Lasagna

Ingredients

Serves 4

For Meat:

1 tablespoon of fresh garlic (minced)

¼ teaspoon of sea salt

½ lbs. ground pork (grass fed)

1 teaspoon of dried oregano

½ lbs. ground beef (grass fed)

1 tablespoon of Italian seasoning

1 cup of onions (diced)

For Zucchini Noodles:

1 tablespoon of sea salt

5 large zucchini

Spice Blend:

½ teaspoon of minced onions

¾ teaspoon of black pepper

½ tablespoon of fresh garlic (minced)

½ teaspoon of red pepper flakes

1 teaspoon of dried parsley

¼ teaspoon of paprika

1 teaspoon of Italian seasoning

¼ teaspoon of fennel seed

1 teaspoon of sea salt

For 'Cheese':

6 tablespoons of water

2 cups of raw cashews (soak in water overnight)

½ teaspoon of garlic powder

2 tablespoons of fresh lemon juice

1 teaspoon of onion powder

Black pepper to taste

1 ¼ teaspoon of sea salt

Others:

½ cup of fresh parsley

¾ cup of crushed tomatoes

¾ cup of tomato sauce

Directions

Pre-heat your oven to 350 degrees F.

Grease a 9 x 13 inch baking dish with olive oil.

Use a mandolin to slice zucchini into 1/8 inch thin slices.

Spread zucchini slices flat on the bottom of 2 cookie sheets.

Sprinkle with salt.

Bake for 15- 25 minutes or until lightly browned.

Combine spice blend ingredients in a bowl. Mix half of the mixture with the pork (in a bowl) and mix well.

Place a saucepan over medium heat.

Place your seasoned ground pork to the pan along with ground beef, garlic and diced onions. Cook until the meat is browned.

Add oregano, pinch of black pepper, Italian seasoning and salt to taste. Continue to cook until meat turns golden brown.

Drain your soaked cashew and pour it in a high-powered blender. Add lemon juice and other cheese ingredients. Process until smooth and set aside.

Combine crushed tomatoes and tomato sauce in a separate bowl. Set aside.

Remove zucchini from oven and transfer to a paper towel. Place another paper towel on it to cover it up. Press it down gently to remove excess moisture.

Pour half of the tomato sauce to the bottom of your greased baking pan. Spread it out evenly.

Add half of the meat mixture to the top.

Layer half of the zucchini noodles on top.

And then half of the 'cheese'

Sprinkle half of the parsley on top.

Repeat the layers.

Bake for 40-45 minutes or until golden brown.

Serve and garnish with fresh parsley.

One-Pan Paleo Bacon Wrapped Chicken

Ingredients

Serves 4

½ teaspoon of sea salt

5 boneless chicken thighs (cut in half)

Black pepper, and fresh thyme or rosemary to taste

10 slices of nitrate and sugar-free bacon

½ teaspoon of smoked paprika

2 teaspoons of onion powder

Directions

Combine onion powder, pepper, salt and smoked paprika in a large bowl.

Add chicken to the bowl and toss so that the spices can coat the chicken thighs.

Place a cast iron skillet over medium heat and let it heat up for a few minutes.

Pre-heat your oven to 400 degrees F.

Use the bacon slices to wrap up each piece of chicken.

Place each piece of wrapped chicken in the skillet with the seam side facing up. Let it brown for 2 minutes.

Flip carefully and let the other side brown for 2 minutes as well.

Transfer the chicken thighs to the oven and cook for 10-15 minutes or until bacons turn crispy.

Serve with potatoes and garnish with fresh herbs.

Chapter 5: Paleo Dinner Recipes

Amore Lamb Chops

Ingredients

Serves 4

2 teaspoons of Primal Palate Amore (a blend of red chili flakes, garlic, parsley, rosemary, basil, thyme, oregano, onion)

8 whole lamb rib chops

1 teaspoon of Himalayan pink salt

Juice of 1 lemon

⅓ cups of extra virgin olive oil

Directions

Combine olive oil, lemon juice and Amore seasoning in a mason jar. Shake well to combine. Pour in a Ziploc bag.

Add lamb chops to the Ziploc bag and seal it up. Massage the chops well to allow the marinade to penetrate the meat. Place it in the refrigerator for 30 minutes.

While the meat is marinating, pre-heat your grill to medium-high heat.

Place lamb chops on a baking sheet and sprinkle some more amore seasoning on it.

Sprinkle Himalayan salt over the lamb chops before placing it on your grill to cook for 12 minutes.

Flip every 3 minutes.

Remove and serve with roasted potatoes.

Fried Plantains

Ingredients

Serves 4

2 tablespoons of ghee

2 medium-sized yellow plantains (peel and slice into ¼ inch rounds)

Fresh lime wedges

Sea salt to taste

Directions

Place a skillet over medium heat and add ghee to heat up.

Add plantains to the skillet in batches. Fry for 2 minutes and flip.

Fry the other side for another 2 minutes.

Serve and sprinkle sea salt over it.

Add lime wedges on the side.

Balsamic Marinated Tomatoes

Ingredients

Serves 4

8 grape tomatoes (halved)

Black pepper to taste

Balsamic vinegar

Sea salt to taste

Directions

Pour enough balsamic vinegar in each tomato halve.

Sprinkle black pepper and sea salt over it.

Allow it to marinate for 24 hours.

Serve.

Mashed Turnips

Ingredients

Serves 4

2 tablespoons of ghee

4 large turnips

Himalayan pink salt

Directions

Wash, peel and cut turnips into small cubes.

Add turnip cubes to a pot and add water. Boil for 15 minutes.

Drain turnips and mash with a fork.

Serve mashed turnips with some ghee on top.

Sprinkle a dash of Himalayan salt on it and enjoy.

With all the above recipes, it may be easy to get confused where you will start. To get you started, the next part will be a 7-day meal plan (using the recipes above) to get you started.

These recipes are just a few examples for you to try.

In time, you will be able to create your own tasty recipes and be able to mix and match to your own liking.

Chapter 6: 7-Day Meal Plan

Day	Breakfast	Snack	Lunch	Snack	Dinner
1	Eggs in Sweet Potato Nests with a glass of Paleo-compliant smoothies	1 handful of nuts	Root Vegetable Bowls with Cinnamon Maple and Tahini Dressing	1 cup of 1 small serving of fruits or homemade fruit juice with a handful of nuts	Amore lamb chops
2	Coconut fruit bowl with a glass of Pale-compliant smoothie	1 handful of nuts	Low-carb Paleo Zucchini Lasagna	1 cup of 1 small serving of fruits or homemade fruit juice with a handful of nuts	Balsamic Marinated Tomatoes
3	Eggs Benedicts in Ham with a glass of Paleo-compliant smoothies	1 handful of nuts	Salad Nicoise	1 cup of 1 small serving of fruits or homemade fruit juice with a handful of nuts	Fried Plantains
4	Salmon and potato pie with a glass of Paleo-compliant smoothies	1 handful of nuts	Crispy One-Pan Paleo Bacon Wrapped	1 cup of 1 small serving of fruits or homemade fruit juice with a handful of nuts	Mashed Turnips
5	Eggs in Sweet Potato Nests with a glass of Paleo-compliant smoothies	1 handful of nuts	Slow-cooker Briskets Taco Bowls	1 cup of 1 small serving of fruits or homemade fruit juice with a handful of nuts	Amore lamb chops

6	Coconut berry bowl with a glass of Paleo-compliant smoothies	1 handful of nuts	Root Vegetable Bowls with Cinnamon Maple and Tahini Dressing	1 cup of 1 small serving of fruits or homemade fruit juice with a handful of nuts	Mashed Turnips
7	Salmon and potato pie with a glass of Paleo-compliant smoothies	1 handful of nuts	Salad Nicoise	1 cup of 1 small serving of fruits or homemade fruit juice with a handful of nuts	Fried Plantains

Conclusion

We have come to the end of the book. Thank you for reading and congratulations for reading until the end.

The Paleo diet is one of the healthiest diets you can ever do because it doesn't involve starving yourself or doing anything outrageous before you achieve your goals.

It is also one of the cheapest diets and most sustainable in the world because you don't have to spend excessively on Paleo products to get your results - all you have to do is to eat natural foods, and that's it. This means you can actually make Paleo eating your way of life for the rest of your life.

I do hope you enjoyed this eBook, if you learned a few things and found it interesting then I would be very grateful if you would consider **leaving me a review** with a few kind words.

Also, if you found it valuable can you please recommend it to others.

Thank you and good luck with your Paleo Diet!

Please don't forget to leave a Review, it would be very much appreciated.